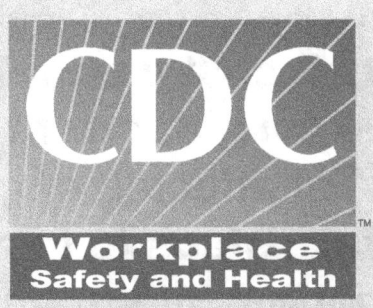

Evaluation of Lead Exposure at an Indoor Firing Range – California

Jessica G. Ramsey, MS, CPE

R. Todd Niemeier, MS, CIH

Health Hazard Evaluation Report
HETA 2008-0275-3146
November 2011

DEPARTMENT OF HEALTH AND HUMAN SERVICES
Centers for Disease Control and Prevention

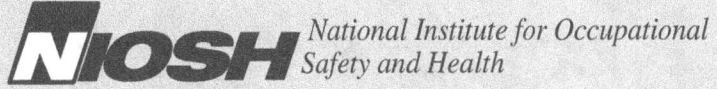 National Institute for Occupational
Safety and Health

The employer shall post a copy of this report for a period of 30 calendar days at or near the workplace(s) of affected employees. The employer shall take steps to insure that the posted determinations are not altered, defaced, or covered by other material during such period. [37 FR 23640, November 7, 1972, as amended at 45 FR 2653, January 14, 1980].

CONTENTS

ABBREVIATIONS

cm	Centimeter
cm^2	Square centimeter
µg/cm^2	Micrograms per square centimeter
µg/dL	Micrograms per deciliter
µg/m^3	Micrograms per cubic meter
µm	Micrometer
mm	Millimeter
ACGIH®	American Conference of Governmental Industrial Hygienists
AIHA	American Industrial Hygiene Association
APF	Assigned protection factor
AL	Action level
BLL	Blood lead level
CDC	Centers for Disease Control and Prevention
CFR	Code of Federal Regulations
CSTE	Council of State and Territorial Epidemiologists
dB	Decibel
DHHS	Department of Health and Human Services
FOH	Federal Occupational Health
fpm	Feet per minute
HEPA	High-efficiency particulate air
HHE	Health hazard evaluation
Hz	Hertz
Lpm	Liters per minute
MDC	Minimum detectable concentration
MERV	Minimum efficiency reporting value
MQC	Minimum quantifiable concentration
NAICS	North American Industry Classification System
ND	Not detected
NIOSH	National Institute for Occupational Safety and Health
OEL	Occupational exposure limit
OSHA	Occupational Safety and Health Administration
PAPR	Powered air purifying respirator
PBZ	Personal breathing zone
PPE	Personal protective equipment
PEL	Permissible exposure limit
REL	Recommended exposure limit
STEL	Short-term exposure limit
TLV®	Threshold limit value
TWA	Time-weighted average
WEEL™	Workplace environmental exposure level
ZPP	Zinc protoporphyrin

The National Institute for Occupational Safety and Health (NIOSH) received a request for a health hazard evaluation at an indoor firing range in California. Employees submitted the request because they were concerned about lead exposures and indoor environmental quality problems during firearms instruction.

What NIOSH Did

- We evaluated the firing range in January 2009 and again in December 2009.

- We looked at the ventilation systems. We also measured airflow in each bay of the firing range.

- We collected personal breathing zone air samples for lead on instructors, shooters, and the hazardous materials technician at the firing range.

- We collected area air samples for lead in the firing range, firearm cleaning area, classroom, lunchroom, and offices.

- We collected floor vacuum samples for lead. Samples were taken from rugs and carpet at the entrance to the firing range and in the firearm cleaning area, lunchroom, armory, and offices.

- We collected surface wipe samples for lead in various locations. We sampled areas in the firing range, firearm cleaning area, classroom, lunchroom, armory, and offices.

- We reviewed medical monitoring results of instructors and the hazardous materials technician.

What NIOSH Found

- Airflow along and downrange of the firing line did not meet the NIOSH recommendations.

- The firing range was dry swept during cleaning.

- Exposures for one instructor, one shooter, and the hazardous materials technician were above the occupational exposure limits for lead for an 8-hour time-weighted average.

- Another shooter's exposure was above the Occupational Safety and Health Administration (OSHA) action level.

- Low concentrations of lead were found in area air samples from the firing range and firearm cleaning area.

- Surface wipe and floor vacuum samples detected lead in various places around the facility.

- Two instructors had threshold shifts that meet the NIOSH definition. Four instructors had slightly more hearing loss in the left ear than the right ear.

What Managers Can Do

- Install a ventilation system that that can deliver the NIOSH-recommended airflow at the firing line and downrange.

- Do not dry sweep the firing range. Clean the floor with an explosion-proof vacuum cleaner with high-efficiency particulate air filters.

- Conduct periodic air sampling. This information will help evaluate whether changes made to the ventilation system and administrative practices have changed lead exposures.

- Remove all carpet in the facility.

- Improve general housekeeping practices, especially in the lunchroom, classroom, and office areas.

- Continue to do medical monitoring. Make sure these activities are done in accordance with the OSHA lead standard.

What Employees Can Do

- Instructors should refrain from using firearms on their workdays.

- Continue to wear dual hearing protection while in the firing range. Dual hearing protection includes ear plugs and earmuffs.

- Wash hands, arms, and face before eating, drinking, or touching others.

- Wear chemical-resistant gloves and tight-fitting goggles when cleaning firearms to protect your skin and eyes from potential chemical hazards.

- Change clothes and shoes before leaving the facility. When possible, also shower before leaving the facility.

- Wash clothes worn in the firing range separately from your family's clothes.

- Report any health concerns to your employer. If needed, seek medical care.

Summary

NIOSH evaluated lead exposures among instructors, shooters, and the hazardous materials technician at an indoor firing range. We found that some exposures exceeded applicable OELs. We also found lead on work surfaces throughout the facility. Recommendations for reducing the risk of lead exposure include installing a new ventilation system that meets NIOSH recommendations for airflow, eliminating dry sweeping, and improving housekeeping practices.

In August 2008, NIOSH received an HHE request from employees at an indoor small arms firing range concerned about lead exposure and indoor environmental quality. We met with employer and employee representatives and observed work processes, practices, and workplace conditions on January 12–13, 2009. We also evaluated the ventilation systems, measured airflow in the firing range, and spoke with employees. On the basis of this initial visit, we recommended installing a new ventilation system capable of delivering the NIOSH-recommended airflow.

The follow-up site visit to collect air and surface lead samples was scheduled for March 2009; however, we delayed this site visit until December 2009 because of plans to install a new ventilation system in the firing range. This renovation was still delayed by the time of the December site visit, so we offered instead to collect air and surface samples to assess lead exposure before and after installation of the new ventilation system. This report only describes conditions before installation of the new ventilation system.

On December 8–10, 2009, we collected PBZ air samples on firing range instructors (instructors), shooters, and the hazardous materials technician at the facility. General area air samples, floor vacuum samples, and surface wipe samples were collected in areas around the facility. We also repeated the airflow measurements in the firing range.

The lead concentrations from PBZ air sampling on instructors ranged from ND–96 $\mu g/m^3$ over the sampling period (calculated 8-hour TWAs were ND–83 $\mu g/m^3$); one instructor's calculated TWA exposure (83 $\mu g/m^3$) exceeded applicable OELs for an 8-hour TWA. For shooters, PBZ lead exposures ranged from 42–340 $\mu g/m^3$ over the sampling periods (calculated 8-hour TWAs were 10–99 $\mu g/m^3$). One shooter who repeated a portion of the qualification had an exposure of 99 $\mu g/m^3$; this exceeded applicable OELs for an 8-hour TWA. The hazardous materials technician's lead exposure was 3,200 $\mu g/m^3$ over the sampling period (calculated 8-hour TWA was 670 $\mu g/m^3$), exceeding the applicable OELs for an 8-hour TWA. The PBZ air sample was collected outside the loose-fitting PAPR that the hazardous materials technician wore while sweeping, vacuuming, and changing exhaust air vent filters in the firing range.

SUMMARY
(CONTINUED)

Floor vacuum and surface wipe sample results showed the presence of lead on work surfaces. This suggests that workplace contamination was being tracked into these areas by employees' footwear, clothing, or hands.

Our review of the instructors' medical monitoring results indicated that BLLs were all below 10 µg/dL of lead. While reviewing medical records, we noted that four instructors had slightly more hearing loss in the left ear than the right ear. Two instructors had threshold shifts that met the NIOSH definition of 15 dB or more at any testing frequency.

In addition to our previous recommendation for a new ventilation system, we recommended eliminating dry sweeping, removing carpeting, and improving general housekeeping practices. We also recommended that instructors not use firearms on their workdays and that all personnel working in the firing range wash their hands, arms, and face before eating, drinking, or touching others. Periodic air sampling for lead should be performed whenever changes are made that affect instructor, shooter, or hazardous materials technician exposures. Management should also continue medical monitoring for personnel at the facility.

Keywords: NAICS 928110 (National Security), lead, CAS# 7439-92-1, Indoor Environmental Quality, IEQ, indoor firing range

INTRODUCTION

NIOSH received an HHE request from employees concerning lead exposure and indoor environmental quality at an indoor firing range in California. NIOSH investigators conducted an initial site visit on January 12–13, 2009. During the site visit we met with employer and employee representatives to discuss the HHE request. We looked at the ventilation systems and measured airflow in the firing range. After the visit, we sent a letter summarizing our findings and providing recommendations for reducing lead exposure at the facility.

We planned to make a follow-up visit to collect air and surface lead samples in March 2009. During a phone conversation we learned that funds for a new ventilation system had been requested. The follow-up visit was postponed until a firm decision was made about funding for the new system. In a subsequent phone call in October 2009, we learned that the ventilation system upgrade still had not begun. At that time, we offered to collect air and surface samples to assess lead exposure before and after installation of the new ventilation system.

We returned to the site on December 8–10, 2009, to assess the lead exposure before the new ventilation system was installed. We collected PBZ air samples, general area air samples, and surface wipe samples for lead. Preliminary findings and recommendations were provided in letters sent in June 2010.

BACKGROUND

The facility was located in a one-story building that consisted of the actual firing range and other spaces including multiple offices and cubicles, lunchroom, classroom, tactical hand-to-hand combat training areas, a firearms cleaning area, and an armory. The firing range had four bays; three bays were used for firearms qualifications, and the fourth bay was constructed as a mockup of a building interior for 360° live fire during Special Weapons and Tactics training. The three bays used for firearms qualifications had eight firing lanes in each bay. Firing lanes were fitted with a swinging arm rest during the January 2009 site visit, but these were not used during qualifications and had been removed by the time of the December 2009 site visit.

The firing range had three ventilation units serving the main section of the range. The ventilation systems for the firing range were separate from the rest of the facility and were designed so air traveled from uprange to downrange (from contaminated to less contaminated areas). Supply air was provided through a perforated metal wall plenum (Figure 1) located approximately 16 feet behind the firing line, except near the entry door where it was approximately 10 feet away (Figure 2).

Two sets of return air vents were located downrange. The first set was approximately 36 feet from the firing line at the ceiling at a height of approximately 10 feet. The second set of vents was behind the bullet trap. Each vent contained MERV 8 Pre Pleat Model 40 Standard Pleated Air Filters. The hazardous materials technician explained that a higher MERV-rated filter was too restrictive and resulted in low exhaust air flow and ventilation system malfunction.

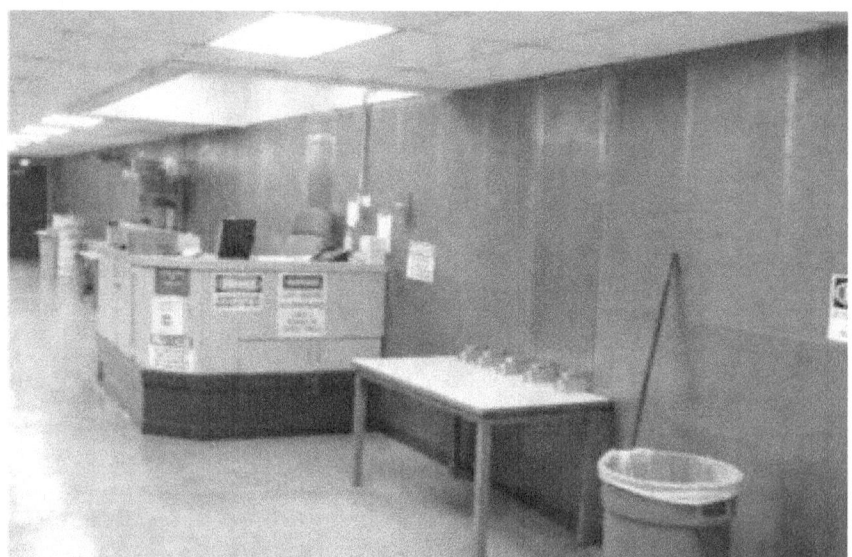

Figure 1. Perforated metal wall plenum and the firing range safety officer's station

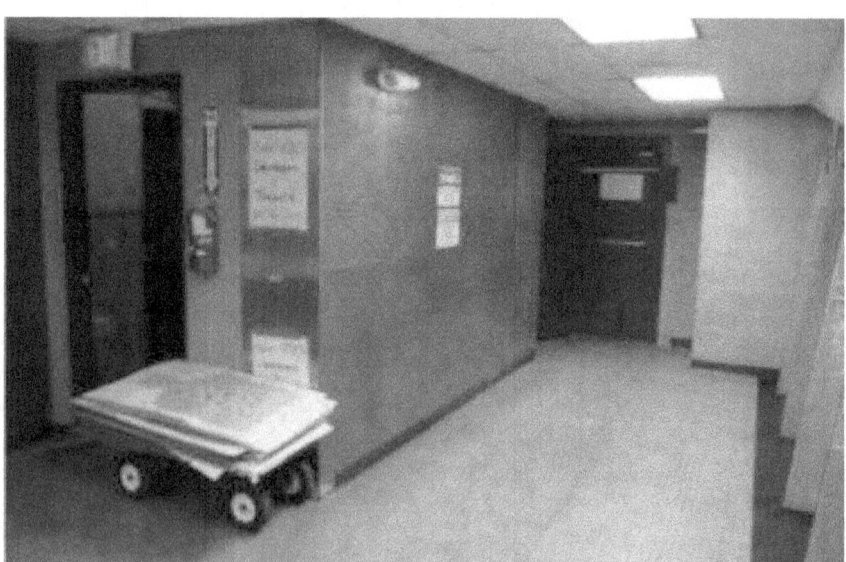

Figure 2. Perforated metal wall plenum near the firing range entry door.

During the January and December 2009 site visits, we measured the rate of airflow in different areas of the firing range. This included measurements at the firing line, below the first set of exhaust air vents, and at the bullet trap. We also noted during both site visits that the firing range was under negative pressure, as desired, in relation to the rest of the facility through the doorway separating these two areas.

During the December 2009 site visit, PBZ air samples for lead were collected on instructors, shooters, and the hazardous materials technician. PBZ air sampling for lead on instructors and shooters was conducted over two days. On December 8, 2009, 20 shooters were qualifying in lanes 5 through 24, and on December 9, 2009, 13 shooters were qualifying in lanes 9 through 21. PBZ air samples were collected on all instructors and on various shooters depending on their lane assignment.

Instructors and shooters were required to wear ear plugs, earmuffs, bulletproof vests, and safety glasses during qualifications. The shooters performed a pistol qualification (72 rounds), a shotgun qualification (5 slugs), a shotgun familiarization (25 rounds of birdshot), and a night pistol practical (48 rounds). Qualifications required both standing and kneeling positions. The total time for all the firearm qualifications was approximately 1 hour. During the firing exercises, the targets were controlled with a pulley system so the shooters did not have to cross the firing line. However, they did cross the line to clean up spent ammunition casings after qualifications were completed. After the qualification exercises, shooters cleaned their firearms for approximately 20 minutes in a cleaning area between the firing range and the classroom area. PBZ air samples were collected on shooters during qualifications and firearm cleaning. Instructors' tasks were varied. If instructors gave the morning lecture, they did not participate in qualifications. If they observed qualifications they also sometimes fired rounds of ammunition.

We collected PBZ air samples on the hazardous materials technician on December 8 and December 9, 2009. The hazardous materials technician was responsible for daily firing range cleanup. This included removal of lead-contaminated debris and dust from the firing range. The hazardous materials technician cleaned the range each morning before qualifications, Monday through Friday. This included dry sweeping the range with a push broom, and then vacuuming the range with a Nilfisk GM80 HEPA vacuum. This

ASSESSMENT (CONTINUED)

procedure was repeated in the space behind the bullet trap. The hazardous materials technician was also responsible for changing the exhaust air vent filters in the firing range and behind the bullet trap (usually three times per week), as well as emptying the bullet trap trough as needed (usually twice per week). The hazardous materials technician wore two pairs of disposable coveralls, butyl rubber gloves, and a loose-fitting PAPR respirator during firing range cleaning and filter change activities. He donned the PPE in the trailer outside the facility. He doffed the outside coveralls inside the back or front of the firing range depending on where he was working. Before he exited the shooting area he wet wiped his PAPR and stepped into the non-shooting area of the range where he doffed the inside coveralls and removed his respirator.

Other lead sampling conducted on December 8–10, 2009, included general area air samples, floor vacuum samples, and surface wipe samples. General area air samples were collected in the firing range, firearm cleaning area, classroom, lunchroom, and offices. Floor vacuum samples for lead content from rugs and carpet were collected in various locations around the facility. Surface wipe samples for lead were collected from various horizontal surfaces around the facility.

Details on the methods for the ventilation system evaluation, as well as air, surface, and vacuum sampling are presented in Appendix A. A discussion of OELs and potential health effects is presented in Appendix B.

We also reviewed medical monitoring results including BLL, ZPP levels, and audiograms performed on instructors from 2007–2011. This monitoring was performed by FOH, under contract with the facility. Annual testing is required per the OSHA lead standard; however FOH is available on-site twice a year in case instructors are on leave one of the two days.

RESULTS

A summary of the ventilation flow rate measurements is provided in Table 1. Airflow along the firing line did not meet the NIOSH-recommended minimum airflow of 50 fpm [NIOSH 2009]. Some of the downrange measures met the NIOSH-recommended minimum airflow of 30 fpm [NIOSH 2009]. The tables in Appendix C provide the air flow rates at specific areas along the firing line in each lane. Tables C1, C2, and C3 provide the supply airflow measurement data that we collected in January 2009 in

RESULTS
(CONTINUED)

each of the three bays used for firearms qualifications. Tables C4, C5, and C6 provide the supply airflow measurement data collected in the same areas in December 2009.

Table 1. Summary of ventilation measurements (fpm) in each bay used for firearms qualification

Date	Location	Firing Line	Downrange First Exhaust Air Vent	Bullet Trap
January 2009	Bay 1: Lanes 1–8	37	27	21
	Bay 2: Lanes 9–16	45	36	18
	Bay 3: Lanes 17–24	38	36	22
December 2009	Bay 1: Lanes 1–8	48	14	14
	Bay 2: Lanes 9–16	36	24	23
	Bay 3: Lanes 17–24	44	38	24

Individual results of the PBZ air sampling for lead on instructors and shooters are presented in Appendix C, Tables C7 and C8. A summary of these results is shown in Table 2. The instructors' lead concentrations ranged from ND–96 $\mu g/m^3$ over the sampling period (86–416 minutes). We did not collect PBZ air samples on instructors during their other work activities outside of the range; however, general area air samples taken in the staff office and lunchroom were ND (Table C9). Assuming that the instructors received no further exposure to airborne lead during that work shift, these results equate to 8-hour TWAs ranging from ND–83 $\mu g/m^3$. One instructor's exposure (83 $\mu g/m^3$) exceeded the OELs of 50 $\mu g/m^3$ for an 8-hour TWA. Under the OSHA general industry lead standard (29 CFR 1910.1025), the PEL for airborne exposure to lead is 50 $\mu g/m^3$ for an 8-hour TWA. The NIOSH REL and ACGIH TLV are also 50 $\mu g/m^3$ for an 8-hour TWA [NIOSH 2010; ACGIH 2011].

Table 2. Concentrations of lead on PBZ air samples of instructors, shooters, and the hazardous materials technician

Title	Sample Time (minutes)	Sample Concentration ($\mu g/m^3$)	8-hour TWA Concentration ($\mu g/m^3$)
Instructors	86–416	ND*–96	ND–83†
Shooters	102–145	42–340	10–99†
Hazardous materials technician	101	3,200	670†

*ND = not detected; below the MDC (0.61 $\mu g/m^3$)

†Exceeds the OSHA PEL of 50 $\mu g/m^3$ for an 8-hour TWA; assumes no exposure for unsampled time during the work shift.

The shooters' lead concentrations ranged from 42–340 $\mu g/m^3$ over the sampling periods (102–145 minutes). We did not collect PBZ air samples on shooters during their classroom time; however, a general area air sample taken in the classroom was ND (Table C9). After the shooters completed the qualifications, they left the firing range facility. Assuming the shooters received no further exposure to airborne lead during the day, these results equate to 8-hour TWAs ranging from 10–99 $\mu g/m^3$.

The result of the PBZ air sampling for lead on the hazardous materials technician is presented in Table 2. Assuming no other lead exposure, this hazardous materials technician's 8-hour TWA lead exposure of 670 $\mu g/m^3$ exceeds the OELs.

Results of the general area air sampling for lead are presented in Table C9 (Appendix C). The lead concentrations ranged from ND–3.6 $\mu g/m^3$. Most results were ND or at a concentration between the MDC and the MQC.

Floor vacuum sample results are presented in Table C10 (Appendix C), and surface wipe sample results are presented in Table C11 (Appendix C). The range of sampling results is shown in Table 3. These results showed the presence of lead on work surfaces outside of the range.

Table 3. Concentrations of lead in floor vacuum and surface wipe samples

Sample Type	Sample Concentration ($\mu g/cm^2$)
Floor vacuum	0.025–0.31
Surface wipe	ND*–2.0

*ND = not detected; below the MDC (0.004 $\mu g/cm^2$).

A summary of the medical monitoring results, obtained from FOH, indicated that instructors' BLLs ranged from < 3–6 $\mu g/dL$ and ZPP levels ranged from 28–56 $\mu g/dL$. A full table of results is presented in Table C12 (Appendix C). FOH also provided audiograms for nine instructors who worked at the facility from 2007–2011. It was noted that four employees had slightly more hearing loss in the left ear than the right ear. Only five instructors had multiple audiograms to compare for threshold shifts; of these two had threshold shifts that met the NIOSH definition of 15 dB or more at any testing frequency. The occupational medicine department of the Naval Training Center provided medical monitoring results for the hazardous materials technician. BLLs for the hazardous materials technician were all at or below 12 $\mu g/dL$, and ZPP levels were in the same range as those for instructors.

Discussion

In 2009, NIOSH issued recommendations on occupational exposure to lead and noise in firing ranges [NIOSH 2009]. The design we evaluated in 2009 did not meet many of the NIOSH recommendations for ventilation design. Most notably, our ventilation measurements indicated that airflow along the firing line in all three bays used for firearms qualifications did not meet the NIOSH-recommended minimum airflow of 50 fpm along the firing line. Many of our downrange measures at both the midrange exhaust air vent and bullet trap were also below the NIOSH-recommended downrange minimum airflow of 30 fpm. During our January 2009 site visit, we observed numerous obstructions including garbage cans, placards, tables, and casing sweepers along the perforated wall supply air plenum. These obstructions reduced uniform air flow across the firing line. We noted during our December 2009 site visit that some of the obstructions had been removed; however, other obstructions remained. Additionally, the range safety officer's station blocked the perforated wall supply air plenum in front of several firing lanes in Bays 2 and 3.

We collected PBZ air samples on instructors during their normal shifts on December 8 and 9, 2009. The results of this evaluation indicate that most instructors had lead exposures that were well below OELs. However, one instructor's exposure exceeded the lead OELs on December 9, 2009. This instructor observed qualifications (similar to other instructors) but also fired approximately 55 rounds of shotgun ammunition during the work shift. This was not typical; however, some instructors did fire their own guns or other guns on various days.

We collected PBZ air samples on shooters while they were performing firearms qualifications and cleaning their firearms. Overall, sampling results for lead for shooters were much higher over the sampling period as compared to instructors. However, because qualification and firearms cleaning only lasted approximately 2–3 hours, most of the shooters' exposures were below 8-hour TWA OELs for lead. However, one shooter's exposure (an 8-hour TWA exposure, 99 µg/m³) was almost two times greater than the OELs for lead on December 8, 2009. This shooter returned to the firing range during the lunch break to repeat some of the qualifications. Another shooter had an 8-hour TWA of 32 µg/m³, which is above the OSHA AL of 30 µg/m³. This shooter was positioned in Lane 16 on December 8, 2009. The ventilation flow rate measurement at Lane 16 during the December site visit was 13 fpm (at 5-foot height), which was the lowest flow rate measured along the firing line. The airflow for Lane 16 may have been obstructed by the range safety officer's station.

The PBZ sample collected on the hazardous materials technician on December 9, 2009, was collected outside the loose-fitting PAPR that he wore during all work activities cleaning the firing range. The hazardous materials technician's lead exposure collected in this sample was greater than 13 times the OELs for lead. In this instance a maximum use concentration for lead over a workday can be calculated by multiplying the loose-fitting PAPR APF (25) and the lead OEL (50 $\mu g/m^3$), equaling 1250 $\mu g/m^3$. If it is assumed the hazardous materials technician had an 8-hour TWA exposure of 670 $\mu g/m^3$ (which is below the maximum use concentration of 1250 $\mu g/m^3$), the loose-fitting PAPR should be protective under these conditions. However, the hazardous materials technician only worked 101 minutes on December 9, 2009. The exposure over this shorter time period is 3,200 $\mu g/m^3$, a concentration that exceeds the maximum use concentration for a loose-fitting PAPR. Therefore, further reductions in exposure are needed. This very high exposure is likely due to dry sweeping instead of vacuuming the firing range floor. The hazardous materials technician preferred sweeping because the firing range vacuum would not remove the larger cardboard pieces that fell to the floor from targets following qualifications. Dry sweeping is not recommended. The hazardous materials technician informed us that he changed the filter on the HEPA vacuum approximately twice a year and changed the bag in the vacuum about once a month.

Airborne lead was detected in very low concentrations in the firing range (at the range safety officer's station) and firearm cleaning area (between 0.61 $\mu g/m^3$ and 1.9 $\mu g/m^3$). However, because airborne lead was detected in the firearm cleaning area this may have been leading to lead contamination in the office, classroom, and lunchroom areas because it was on the office side of the ventilation system. Lead from contaminated surfaces can be transferred to the skin, especially the hands. This can result in lead ingestion while handling food, beverages, and other items that contact the mouth.

Floor vacuum and surface wipe sample results showed the presence of lead on work surfaces. This suggests that workplace contamination could also be tracked into these areas by employees' footwear, clothing, or hands. Carpeting, which was noted in the lunchroom and staff offices, is not recommended inside a firing range or in rooms adjacent to the range [NIOSH 2009]. No occupational exposure guidelines or regulations exist for lead concentrations on work surfaces; however, lead-contaminated surfaces in the workplace represent a potential source of exposure for employees. OSHA specifies in its substance-specific standard for lead that all surfaces be maintained as free as practicable of accumulations of lead [29 CFR 1910.1025(h)(1)]. Our evaluation showed the highest amount of lead on the armory shelving unit and the top of the filing cabinet near the firearm cleaning area. These two locations are probably rarely cleaned. However, lead was also detected on the top of the modular cabinet in the lunchroom and in the office areas; this indicates that general cleaning needs to be improved throughout the facility.

OSHA's lead standard requires each employer who operates a firing range to determine if any workers may be exposed to lead at or above the AL (30 μg/m^3 as an 8-hour TWA). Worker exposure is defined as exposure that would occur if the workers were not using a respirator. On the basis of our air sampling, instructors, shooters, and the hazardous materials technician may be exposed at the AL, and therefore monitoring their exposure to lead should be performed periodically to ensure continued effectiveness of current protection measures. Additionally, any changes in work practices, equipment, or maintenance procedures would also trigger a need for air sampling.

Because some airborne exposures to lead were identified above the OSHA PEL, the facility should follow OSHA lead regulations to prevent spread of lead contamination outside of the workplace. The regulations (29 CFR 1910.1025) include mandating that employees take showers before leaving the facility and providing locker space to ensure that street clothes are not contaminated with lead dust.

The OSHA lead standard also requires participation in a medical clearance program for lead. Currently, instructors and the hazardous materials technician undergo annual medical monitoring. Our review showed that monitoring results for instructors did not exceed the guideline of 10 μg/dL for BLL recommended by the Association of Occupational and Environmental Clinics [CSTE 2009]. However, the hazardous materials technician exceeded this guideline on 3 occasions with levels up to 12 μg/dL. The hazardous materials technician also participated in a respiratory protection program that met the requirements of the OSHA respiratory protection standard.

DISCUSSION (CONTINUED)

Typically, workers with noise-induced hearing loss have an approximately equal loss in both ears. Our review of the audiograms for instructors showed more hearing loss in the left ear compared to the right ear. Asymmetrical hearing loss is known to occur in shooters [Prosser et al. 1988; Sataloff and Sataloff 2006] and is thought to be related to the person's head position when using firearms such as rifles or shotguns. Right-handed shooters are more likely to have hearing loss in their left ear and left-handed shooters tend to have more hearing loss in their right ear. Although asymmetric hearing loss is more common in shooters than other workers exposed to noise, instructors should be evaluated by an audiologist or ear, nose, and throat specialist to rule out other medical causes for asymmetric loss.

NIOSH defines a hearing threshold shift as a 15-dB change in hearing threshold in any of the audiometric test frequencies. Analysis of the audiograms was limited because several of the instructors only had one or two audiograms available for review. However, of those that we were able to compare, most of the shifts were at 4,000 Hz and 6,000 Hz and differences ranged between 15 dB and 50 dB.

CONCLUSIONS

The results of this evaluation indicated that instructors, shooters, and the hazardous materials technician were exposed to lead above the OELs. In particular, instructors were found to have higher exposure to lead if they used firearms on the days that they observed qualifications. Shooters were found to have higher exposure to lead if they returned to the firing range for additional rounds of shooting. The hazardous materials technician was found to have high levels of exposure to lead which we believe is due to dry sweeping the firing range. Floor vacuum and surface wipe sample results showed the presence of lead on work surfaces throughout the facility. This suggests that workplace contamination is being tracked into these areas by employees' footwear, clothing, or hands. Engineering and administrative controls are recommended to reduce exposures.

On the basis of our findings, we recommend the actions listed below to create a more healthful workplace. We encourage the firing range to use a labor-management health and safety committee or working group to discuss the recommendations in this report and develop an action plan. Those involved in the work can best set priorities and assess the feasibility of our recommendations for the specific situation at the facility. Our recommendations are based on the hierarchy of controls approach (refer to Appendix B: Occupational Exposure Limits and Health Effects). This approach groups actions by their likely effectiveness in reducing or removing hazards. In most cases, the preferred approach is to eliminate hazardous materials or processes and install engineering controls to reduce exposure or shield employees. Until such controls are in place, or if they are not effective or feasible, administrative measures and/or personal protective equipment may be needed. Most of these recommendations were taken from the NIOSH Alert, "Preventing Occupational Exposures to Lead and Noise at Indoor Firing Ranges" [NIOSH 2009].

Elimination and Substitution

Elimination or substitution of a toxic/hazardous process material is a highly effective means for reducing hazards. Incorporating this strategy into the design or development phase of a project, commonly referred to, as "prevention through design," is most effective because it reduces the need for additional controls in the future.

1. Use non-lead primers designed specifically for firing ranges. Cartridges already loaded with non-lead primers are commercially available for the most popular calibers.

2. Investigate the use of electronic simulation systems using firearms equipped with lasers, which can provide an alternative solution for training new recruits in effective firearm handling and marksmanship without using live ammunition.

Engineering Controls

Engineering controls reduce exposures to employees by removing the hazard from the process or placing a barrier between the hazard and the employee. Engineering controls are very effective at protecting employees without placing primary responsibility of implementation on the employee.

1. Install a ventilation system capable of delivering the NIOSH-recommended airflow at the firing line and downrange. Airflow along the firing line should be no more than 75 fpm with a minimum acceptable flow of 50 fpm. To minimize fallout of firearm emissions downrange of the firing line (if desired), downrange airflow should be maintained at a minimum of 30 fpm and should be evenly distributed.

2. Enclose the firearm cleaning area, as airborne lead was detected in this area. This will help to reduce the spread of airborne lead contamination to other areas of the building. Assistance of a contractor familiar with firing range design is strongly encouraged.

3. Remove objects (e.g., cabinets, tables, placards, brass collectors, and garbage cans) obstructing airflow between the supply air inlets and the firing line so that the supply air is distributed uniformly across the width of the firing range.

4. Use HEPA filters or filters with a MERV rating of 18–19 in the exhaust ventilation system.

5. Change filters according to the static pressure guidelines provided by the manufacturer. Filter end-of-service life is indicated by a high-pressure drop across the filter bank. Because pre-filters are the first to encounter contaminated exhaust air from the firing range, they will load fastest. Therefore, pre-filters require more frequent change-outs than high efficiency filters.

Administrative Controls

Administrative controls are management-dictated work practices and policies to reduce or prevent exposures to workplace hazards. The effectiveness of administrative changes in work practices for controlling workplace hazards is dependent on management commitment and employee acceptance. Regular monitoring and reinforcement are necessary to ensure that control policies and procedures are not circumvented in the name of convenience or production.

1. Advise instructors to refrain from using firearms on their workdays. If instructors need to use firearms on days when they are observing qualifications, then respiratory protection may be necessary. Confirm these exposures with additional PBZ air sampling.

RECOMMENDATIONS
(CONTINUED)

2. Clean the floor of the firing range thoroughly with an explosion-proof HEPA vacuum cleaner designed to collect lead dust. Dry sweeping should never be used in the firing range. The OSHA general industry lead standard [29 CFR 1910.1025(h)(2)(ii)] states that shoveling, dry or wet sweeping, and brushing may be used only where vacuuming or other equally effective methods have been tried and found ineffective.

3. All personnel should wash their hands, forearms, and faces before eating, drinking, or having any hand contact with the face or with other people.

4. Avoid skin contact with spent cartridges whenever possible. Wear disposable gloves should when removing larger objects that cannot be removed with a HEPA vacuum cleaner.

5. Clean floor and horizontal surfaces inside the firing range routinely with a detergent. U.S. Environmental Protection Agency studies show that general all-purpose cleaners are adequate for both general cleaning and post-intervention cleaning.

6. Remove carpeting in rooms adjacent to the firing range. Accumulation of lead dust in carpets is a health hazard, and accumulation of unspent primer in carpets is a fire hazard.

7. Improve general housekeeping practices throughout the facility to keep horizontal surfaces free of dust and debris. Lunchroom, classroom, and office areas should receive special attention because of the potential for lead exposure through hand-to-mouth contact. Detergents that contain trisodium phosphate are best for cleaning surfaces that may have lead contamination.

8. Advise shooters who use a kneeling position on lead contaminated surfaces to place a sheet of paper or other disposable material on the ground beneath them to minimize accumulation of leaded dust on their outer garments.

9. Instruct shooters and instructors to shower, whenever possible, and change clothes at the facility after shooting or performing maintenance or cleaning activities in the firing range. Clothes worn at the firing range should be washed separately from family's clothes.

10. Provide clean change rooms for employees who work in areas where there is airborne exposure to lead. Also provide workers with two lockers to allow them to separate street clothes from lead-contaminated work clothes.

11. Leave shoes worn on the firing range at the range or bag them before leaving the range to prevent lead from being tracked into cars and onto home floors and carpets. As an alternative, use step-off cleaning pads at the exit of the firing range to help reduce the amount of lead contamination on shoes. Disposable shoe coverings can also be used while firing and cleaning, then discarded upon leaving the range.

Worker Exposure and Medical Health Monitoring

Instructors and the hazardous materials technician had medical monitoring performed annually. Our results indicate that instructors, shooters, and the hazardous materials technician may be exposed above the OSHA AL for lead; therefore, the following recommendations are provided.

1. Perform periodic air sampling for lead whenever changes are made that affect instructor, shooter, or hazardous materials technician exposures. If instructors or shooters continue to have exposures above the OELs due to increased time spent using firearms, then respiratory protection would be required. Once dry sweeping is eliminated and a new cleaning procedure is in place, repeat air sampling on the hazardous materials technician to determine exposure levels and what level of respiratory protection is needed.

2. Conduct air sampling under the direction of a certified industrial hygienist or other safety and health professional with appropriate training and expertise.

3. Perform wipe sampling regularly on surfaces in the firing range. Wipe samples can provide information about how well these surfaces are being cleaned, whether lead is being transported from the firing range to other parts of the facility, and about the potential for lead exposure.

4. Follow the OSHA general industry lead standard, which contains provisions for the medical monitoring of workers exposed to lead [29 CFR 1910.1025(j)]. NIOSH supports using these provisions for firing range workers.

5. Report any symptoms consistent with lead exposure in adults to the employer or firing range safety officer. Common symptoms of lead poisoning in adults include nausea, diarrhea, vomiting, poor appetite, weight loss, anemia, excess lethargy or hyperactivity, headaches, abdominal pain, and kidney problems.

Personal Protective Equipment

PPE is the least effective means for controlling employee exposures. Proper use of PPE requires a comprehensive program, and calls for a high level of employee involvement and commitment to be effective. The use of PPE requires the choice of the appropriate equipment to reduce the hazard and the development of supporting programs such as training, change-out schedules, and medical assessment if needed. PPE should not be relied upon as the sole method for limiting employee exposures. Rather, PPE should be used until engineering and administrative controls can be demonstrated to be effective in limiting exposures to acceptable levels.

1. Encourage personnel cleaning firearms to use chemical-resistant gloves and tight-fitting goggles for skin and eye protection against potential chemical hazards. Firing range operators should provide specific guidance about proper and appropriate use of skin and eye protection.

2. Select respirators based on their APF, considering the PBZ lead exposures of instructors and the hazardous materials technician. Respirator type should be reconsidered whenever changes are made that affect exposures.

3. Continue to require instructors and shooters to wear dual hearing protection (ear plugs and earmuffs) while in the firing range. For maximum protection, select earmuffs and ear plugs that provide a high level of noise attenuation. To ensure that hearing protectors have adequate noise attenuation and are worn correctly, perform fit testing. Some hearing protection manufacturers are able to conduct hearing protection fit testing. Additionally, because of the critical importance of proper fit, the firing range safety officer should regularly check to ensure that hearing protection is worn correctly.

REFERENCES

ACGIH [2011]. 2011 TLVs® and BEIs®: threshold limit values for chemical substances and physical agents and biological exposure indices. Cincinnati, OH: American Conference of Governmental Industrial Hygienists.

CSTE [2009]. Public health reporting and national notification for elevated blood lead levels. CSTE position statement 09-OH-02. Atlanta: CSTE 2009 [http://www.cste.org/ps2009/09-OH-02.pdf]. Date accessed: October 2011.

CFR. Code of Federal Regulations. Washington, DC: U.S. Government Printing Office, Federal Register.

NIOSH [2009]. NIOSH alert: preventing occupational exposures to lead and noise at indoor firing ranges. Cincinnati, OH: U.S. Department of Health and Human Services, Centers for Disease Control and Prevention, National Institute for Occupational Safety and Health, DHHS (NIOSH) Publication No. 2009-136.

NIOSH [2010]. NIOSH pocket guide to chemical hazards. Cincinnati, OH: U.S. Department of Health and Human Services, Centers for Disease Control and Prevention, National Institute for Occupational Safety and Health, DHHS (NIOSH) Publication No. 2010-168c. [http://www.cdc.gov/niosh/npg/]. Date accessed: October 2011.

Prosser S, Tartari M, Arslan E [1988]. Hearing loss in sports hunters exposed to occupational noise. Br J Aud 22(2):85–91.

Sataloff R, Sataloff J [2006]. Occupational hearing loss. 3rd ed. Boca Raton, FL: Taylor and Francis Group, LLC, pp. 411–440.

APPENDIX A: METHODS

Ventilation Measurements

A TSI VelociCalc® Plus air velocity meter, model 8386A (TSI, Inc, Shoreview, Minnesota) was used to measure airflow at different locations within the firing range, including at the firing line, at the first set of exhaust air vents (located 36 feet downrange from the firing line), and at the bullet trap. Triplicate measurements were collected in each lane along the firing lane at two different heights (approximately 3 feet and 5 feet). These measurements were averaged together and reported for each location along the firing lane.

Air Sampling for Lead

Air samples for lead were collected on 37-mm diameter, 0.8-µm pore size mixed cellulose ester filters using SKC Air Check® 2000 air sampling pumps (SKC, Inc, Eighty Four, Pennsylvania) calibrated at a flow rate of 2 Lpm. The inlet port of the sampling pump was connected to the sampling media with Tygon® tubing. For PBZ air samples, the sampling media was attached to the employee's lapel within the breathing zone, roughly defined as an area in front of the shoulders with a radius of 6 to 9 inches. The general area air samples were placed throughout the facility including areas where instructors or shooters took breaks and ate lunch. Air samples were analyzed by inductively coupled argon plasma-atomic emission spectroscopy according to NIOSH Method 7303 [NIOSH 2011].

Surface Wipe Sampling for Lead

Surface wipe samples were collected with premoistened Palintest® Dust Wipes (Palintest USA, Erlanger, Kentucky) according to NIOSH Method 9102 [NIOSH 2011]. The collection procedure was as follows: (1) identify the area to be sampled; (2) put on a pair of disposable nitrile gloves; (3) place the wipe flat on the surface as defined by the 10 cm by 10 cm (100 cm² area) disposable template and wipe the surface using three to four horizontal S-strokes, side-to-side so that the entire surface is covered; (4) fold the exposed side of the wipe in and wipe the area with three or four vertical S-strokes; (5) fold the wipe once more and wipe the area with three or four horizontal S-strokes; and (6) fold the pad, exposed side in, and place in a sterile container. A new template and a pair of disposable gloves were used for each surface wipe sample. The surface wipe samples were digested and analyzed by inductively coupled argon plasma-atomic emission spectroscopy according to NIOSH Method 9102 with modifications [NIOSH 2011].

Vacuum Sampling for Lead

Vacuum samples were collected on 37-mm diameter, 0.8-µm pore size mixed cellulose ester filters with small nozzle attachments connected to SKC Air Check® 2000 air sampling pumps (SKC, Inc, Eighty Four, Pennsylvania) calibrated at a flow rate of 2 Lpm. The surface was vacuumed in the same way other surfaces were wiped, three sets of S-curve wipes over a 100 cm² area determined by a disposable template according to NIOSH Method 9102 [NIOSH 2011]. These samples were also analyzed by inductively coupled argon plasma-atomic emission spectroscopy according to NIOSH Method 7303 [NIOSH 2011].

Reference

NIOSH [2011]. NIOSH manual of analytical methods (NMAM®). 4th ed. Schlecht PC, O'Connor PF, eds. Cincinnati, OH: U.S. Department of Health and Human Services, Centers for Disease Control and Prevention, National Institute for Occupational Safety and Health, DHHS (NIOSH) Publication 94-113 (August 1994); 1st Supplement Publication 96-135, 2nd Supplement Publication 98-119; 3rd Supplement 2003-154. [http://www.cdc.gov/niosh/nmam/].

In evaluating the hazards posed by workplace exposures, NIOSH investigators use both mandatory (legally enforceable) and recommended OELs for chemical, physical, and biological agents as a guide for making recommendations. OELs have been developed by federal agencies and safety and health organizations to prevent the occurrence of adverse health effects from workplace exposures. Generally, OELs suggest levels of exposure that most employees may be exposed to for up to 10 hours per day, 40 hours per week, for a working lifetime, without experiencing adverse health effects. However, not all employees will be protected from adverse health effects even if their exposures are maintained below these levels. A small percentage may experience adverse health effects because of individual susceptibility, a preexisting medical condition, and/or a hypersensitivity (allergy). In addition, some hazardous substances may act in combination with other workplace exposures, the general environment, or with medications or personal habits of the employee to produce adverse health effects even if the occupational exposures are controlled at the level set by the exposure limit. Also, some substances can be absorbed by direct contact with the skin and mucous membranes in addition to being inhaled, which contributes to the individual's overall exposure.

Most OELs are expressed as a TWA exposure. A TWA refers to the average exposure during a normal 8- to 10-hour workday. Some chemical substances and physical agents have recommended STEL or ceiling values where adverse health effects are caused by exposures over a short period. Unless otherwise noted, the STEL is a 15-minute TWA exposure that should not be exceeded at any time during a workday, and the ceiling limit is an exposure that should not be exceeded at any time.

In the United States, OELs have been established by federal agencies, professional organizations, state and local governments, and other entities. Some OELs are legally enforceable limits, while others are recommendations. The U.S. Department of Labor OSHA PELs (29 CFR 1910 [general industry]; 29 CFR 1926 [construction industry]; and 29 CFR 1917 [maritime industry]) are legal limits enforceable in workplaces covered under the Occupational Safety and Health Act of 1970. NIOSH RELs are recommendations based on a critical review of the scientific and technical information available on a given hazard and the adequacy of methods to identify and control the hazard. NIOSH RELs can be found in the *NIOSH Pocket Guide to Chemical Hazards* [NIOSH 2010]. NIOSH also recommends different types of risk management practices (e.g., engineering controls, safe work practices, employee education/ training, personal protective equipment, and exposure and medical monitoring) to minimize the risk of exposure and adverse health effects from these hazards. Other OELs that are commonly used and cited in the United States include the TLVs recommended by ACGIH, a professional organization, and the WEELs recommended by the American Industrial Hygiene Association, another professional organization. The TLVs and WEELs are developed by committee members of these associations from a review of the published, peer-reviewed literature. They are not consensus standards. ACGIH TLVs are considered voluntary exposure guidelines for use by industrial hygienists and others trained in this discipline "to assist in the control of health hazards" [ACGIH 2011]. WEELs have been established for some chemicals "when no other legal or authoritative limits exist" [AIHA 2011].

Outside the United States, OELs have been established by various agencies and organizations and include both legal and recommended limits. The Institut für Arbeitsschutz der Deutschen Gesetzlichen Unfallversicherung (IFA, Institute for Occupational Safety and Health of the German Social Accident Insurance) maintains a database of international OELs from European Union member states, Canada

(Québec), Japan, Switzerland, and the United States. The database, available at http://www.dguv.de/ifa/en/gestis/limit_values/index.jsp, contains international limits for over 1,500 hazardous substances and is updated periodically.

Employers should understand that not all hazardous chemicals have specific OSHA PELs, and for some agents the legally enforceable and recommended limits may not reflect current health-based information. However, an employer is still required by OSHA to protect its employees from hazards even in the absence of a specific OSHA PEL. OSHA requires an employer to furnish employees a place of employment free from recognized hazards that cause or are likely to cause death or serious physical harm [Occupational Safety and Health Act of 1970 (Public Law 91–596, sec. 5(a)(1))]. Thus, NIOSH investigators encourage employers to make use of other OELs when making risk assessments and risk management decisions to best protect the health of their employees. NIOSH investigators also encourage the use of the traditional hierarchy of controls approach to eliminate or minimize identified workplace hazards. This includes, in order of preference, the use of (1) substitution or elimination of the hazardous agent, (2) engineering controls (e.g , local exhaust ventilation, process enclosure, dilution ventilation), (3) administrative controls (e.g., limiting time of exposure, employee training, work practice changes, medical surveillance), and (4) personal protective equipment (e.g., respiratory protection, gloves, eye protection, hearing protection). Control banding, a qualitative risk assessment and risk management tool, is a complementary approach to protecting employee health that focuses resources on exposure controls by describing how a risk needs to be managed. Information on control banding is available at http://www.cdc.gov/niosh/topics/ctrlbanding/. This approach can be applied in situations where OELs have not been established or can be used to supplement the OELs, when available.

Below we provide the OELs and surface contamination limits as well as a discussion of the potential health effects for exposure to lead.

Lead

Lead is ubiquitous in U.S. urban environments because of the widespread use of lead compounds in industry, gasoline, and paints during the past century. Exposure to lead occurs via inhalation of dust and fume and via ingestion through contact with lead-contaminated hands, food, cigarettes, and clothing. Absorbed lead accumulates in the body in the soft tissues and bones. Lead is stored in bones for decades, and may cause health effects long after exposure as it is slowly released in the body.

Symptoms of chronic lead poisoning include headache, joint and muscle aches, weakness, fatigue, irritability, depression, constipation, anorexia, and abdominal discomfort [Moline and Landrigan 2005]. Overexposure to lead may also result in kidney damage, anemia, high blood pressure, infertility and reduced sex drive in both sexes, and impotence. In most cases, an individual's BLL is a good indication of recent exposure to lead, with a half-life (the time interval it takes for the quantity in the body to be reduced by half its initial value) of 1–2 months [Lauwerys and Hoet 2001; Moline and Landrigan 2005; NCEH 2005]. Elevated ZPP levels have also been used as an indicator of chronic lead intoxication; however, other factors, such as iron deficiency, can cause an elevated ZPP level, so the BLL is a more specific test for evaluating occupational lead exposure.

Under the OSHA general industry lead standard (29 CFR 1910.1025), the PEL for airborne exposure to lead is 50 µg/m³ for an 8-hour TWA. The standard requires lowering the PEL for shifts exceeding 8 hours, medical monitoring for employees exposed to airborne lead at or above the AL of 30 µg/m³ (8-hour TWA), medical removal of employees whose average BLL is 50 µg/dL or greater, and economic protection for medically removed workers. Medically removed workers cannot return to jobs involving lead exposure until their BLL is below 40 µg/dL. NIOSH has an REL for lead of 50 µg/m³ averaged over an 8-hour work shift [NIOSH 2010]. ACGIH has a TLV for lead of 50 µg/m³ (8-hour TWA), with worker BLLs to be controlled to or below 30 µg/dL, and designation of lead as an animal carcinogen [ACGIH 2011].

The NIOSH REL is consistent with the OSHA PEL, which is intended to maintain worker BLLs below 40 µg/dL. This is also intended to prevent overt symptoms of lead poisoning, but is not sufficient to protect workers from more subtle adverse health effects like hypertension, renal dysfunction, and reproductive and cognitive effects [Schwartz and Stewart 2007; Schwartz and Hu 2007; Brown-Williams et al. 2009]. Adverse effects on the adult reproductive, cardiovascular, and hematologic systems, and on the development of children of exposed workers, can occur at BLLs as low as 10 µg/dL [Sussell 1998]. Recommendations from the March 2007 edition of Environmental Health Perspectives' Mini-Monograph on adult lead exposure and from the Association of Occupational and Environmental Clinics include advising workers and shooters that BLLs should be kept below 10 µg/dL [CSTE 2009].

In homes with a family member occupationally exposed to lead, care must be taken to prevent "take home" of lead, that is, lead carried into the home on clothing, skin, hair, and in vehicles. High BLLs in resident children and elevated concentrations of lead in the house dust have been found in the homes of workers employed in industries associated with high lead exposure [Grandjean and Bach 1986]. Particular effort should be made to ensure that children of persons who work in areas of high lead exposure receive a BLL test. The current CDC screening guidelines for children use 10 µg/dL as a "level of concern" in order to intervene and prevent long-term cognitive deficits [CDC 2005].

Lead-contaminated surface dust represents a potential source of lead exposure, particularly for young children. This may occur either by direct hand-to-mouth contact, or indirectly from hand-to-mouth contact with contaminated clothing, cigarettes, or food. Previous studies have found a significant correlation between resident children's BLLs and house dust lead levels [Farfel and Chisholm 1990]. In the workplace, generally there is little or no correlation between surface lead levels and employee exposures because ingestion exposures are highly dependent on personal hygiene practices and available facilities for maintaining personal hygiene. No current federal standard provides a permissible limit for lead contamination of surfaces in occupational settings.

References

ACGIH [2011]. 2011 TLVs® and BEIs®: threshold limit values for chemical substances and physical agents and biological exposure indices. Cincinnati, OH: American Conference of Governmental Industrial Hygienists.

AIHA [2011]. AIHA 2011 Emergency response planning guidelines (ERPG) & workplace environmental exposure levels (WEEL) handbook. Fairfax, VA: American Industrial Hygiene Association.

Brown-Williams H, Lichterman J, Kosnett M [2009]. Indecent exposure: lead puts workers and families at risk. Health Research in Action, University of California, Berkeley. Perspectives 4(1)1-9.

CDC [2005]. Preventing lead poisoning in young children. Atlanta: Centers for Disease Control and Prevention. [http://www.cdc.gov/nceh/lead/publications/prevleadpoisoning.pdf]. Date accessed: October 2011.

CFR. Code of Federal Regulations. Washington, DC: U.S. Government Printing Office, Federal Register.

CSTE [2009]. Public health reporting and national notification for elevated blood lead levels. CSTE position statement 09-OH-02. Atlanta: Council of State and Territorial Epidemiologists [http://www.cste.org/ps2009/09-OH-02.pdf]. Date accessed: October 2011.

Farfel MR, Chisholm JJ [1990]. Health and environmental outcomes of traditional and modified practices for abatement of residential lead-based paint. Am J Pub Health 80(10):1240-1245.

Grandjean P, Bach E [1986]. Indirect exposures: the significance of bystanders at work and at home. Am Ind Hyg Assoc J 47(12):819-824.

Lauwerys RR, Hoet P [2001]. Biological monitoring of exposure to inorganic and organometallic substances. In: Industrial chemical exposure: guidelines for biological monitoring. 3rd ed. Boca Raton, FL: CRC Press, LLC, pp. 21-180.

Moline JM, Landrigan PJ [2005]. Lead. In: Textbook of clinical occupational and environmental medicine. Rosenstock L, Cullen MR, Brodkin CA, Redlich CA, eds. 2nd ed. Philadelphia, PA: Elsevier Saunders, pp. 967-979.

NCEH [2005]. Third national report on human exposure to environmental chemicals. Atlanta, GA: U.S. Department of Health and Human Services, Centers for Disease Control and Prevention. National Center for Environmental Health Publication No. 05-0570.

NIOSH [2009]. NIOSH alert: preventing occupational exposures to lead and noise at indoor firing ranges. Cincinnati, OH: U.S. Department of Health and Human Services, Centers for Disease Control and Prevention, National Institute for Occupational Safety and Health, DHHS (NIOSH) Publication No. 2009-136.

NIOSH [2010]. NIOSH pocket guide to chemical hazards. Cincinnati, OH: U.S. Department of Health and Human Services, Centers for Disease Control and Prevention, National Institute for Occupational Safety and Health, DHHS (NIOSH) Publication No. 2010-168c. [http://www.cdc.gov/niosh/npg/]. Date accessed: October 2011.

Schwartz BS, Hu H [2007]. Adult lead exposure: time for change. Environ Health Perspect 115(3):451–454.

Schwartz BS, Stewart WF [2007]. Lead and cognitive function in adults: a question and answers approach to a review of the evidence for cause, treatment, and prevention. Int Rev Psychiatry 19(6):671–692.

Sussell A [1998]. Protecting workers exposed to lead-based paint hazards: a report to Congress. Cincinnati, OH: U.S. Department of Health and Human Services, Centers for Disease Control and Prevention, National Institute for Occupational Safety and Health, DHHS (NIOSH) Publication No. 98–112.

Appendix C: Tables

Table C1. Bay 1 ventilation flow rates (fpm) measured on January 13, 2009

Firing Lane #	Firing Line		First Exhaust Air Vent		Bullet Trap	
	(~3 feet*)	(~5 feet*)	(~3 feet*)	(~5 feet*)	(~3 feet*)	(~5 feet*)
1	100	40	15	20	10	15
2	10	2	10	30	5	5
3	50	20	10	30	15	20
4	25	40	20	20	30	30
5	40	30	40	20	30	30
6	70	25	30	30	30	40
7	100	10	20	60	10	40
8	20	15	50	30	1	30
Average	52	23	24	30	16	26
Total average	37		27		21	
Total downrange average			24			

* Height at which the rate of airflow was measured.

Table C2. Bay 2 ventilation flow rates (fpm) measured on January 13, 2009

Firing Lane #	Firing Line		First Exhaust Air Vent		Bullet Trap	
	(~3 feet*)	(~5 feet*)	(~3 feet*)	(~5 feet*)	(~3 feet*)	(~5 feet*)
9	60	20	50	40	3	20
10	80	40	30	20	3	30
11	60	20	40	40	10	30
12	80	50	40	60	10	30
13	70	35	40	40	25	30
14	50	10	40	30	10	10
15	70	0	20	30	30	30
16	30	40	30	25	2	20
Average	63	27	36	35	12	25
Total average	45		36		18	
Total downrange average			27			

* Height at which the rate of airflow was measured.

Table C3. Bay 3 ventilation flow rates (fpm) measured on January 13, 2009

Firing Lane #	Firing Line		First Exhaust Air Vent		Bullet Trap	
	(~3 feet*)	(~5 feet*)	(~3 feet*)	(~5 feet*)	(~3 feet*)	(~5 feet*)
17	10	50	40	30	30	20
18	80	30	50	50	30	40
19	60	30	60	30	30	30
20	30	40	50	40	20	10
21	25	25	40	10	10	5
22	60	40	40	20	5	5
23	40	30	30	20	10	10
24	30	30	30	30	60	30
Average	42	34	43	29	24	19
Total average	38		36		22	
Total downrange average			29			

* Height at which the rate of airflow was measured.

Table C4. Bay 1 ventilation flow rates (fpm) measured on December 10, 2009

Firing Lane #	Firing Line		First Exhaust Air Vent		Bullet Trap	
	(~3 feet*)	(~5 feet*)	(~3 feet*)	(~5 feet*)	(~3 feet*)	(~5 feet*)
1	32	52	33	9	20	12
2	39	29	16	10	11	8
3	56	102	19	8	41	11
4	46	96	21	13	6	10
5	53	55	10	10	13	20
6	27	64	19	20	3	21
7	8	53	4	13	17	7
8	8	47	6	8	13	8
Average	34	63	16	11	16	12
Total average	48		14		14	
Total downrange average			14			

* Height at which the rate of airflow was measured.

Appendix C: Tables
(continued)

Table C5. Bay 2 ventilation flow rates (fpm) measured on December 10, 2009

Firing Lane #	Firing Line		First Exhaust Air Vent		Bullet Trap	
	(~3 feet*)	(~5 feet*)	(~3 feet*)	(~5 feet*)	(~3 feet*)	(~5 feet*)
9	16	26	52	6	34	13
10	41	28	35	4	14	18
11	18	17	61	16	57	31
12	41	23	23	14	45	18
13	43	34	12	37	25	11
14	51	46	10	14	26	10
15	72	25	27	24	32	17
16	85	13	23	25	6	9
Average	46	26	30	18	30	16
Total average	36		24		23	
Total downrange average			24			

* Height at which the rate of airflow was measured.

Table C6. Bay 3 ventilation flow rates (fpm) measured on December 10, 2009

Firing Lane #	Firing Line		First Exhaust Air Vent		Bullet Trap	
	(~3 feet*)	(~5 feet*)	(~3 feet*)	(~5 feet*)	(~3 feet*)	(~5 feet*)
17	29	21	59	46	29	13
18	64	14	35	17	41	9
19	63	26	41	8	15	12
20	50	48	40	7	34	12
21	52	51	64	26	42	39
22	49	55	69	23	24	29
23	39	28	51	39	14	14
24	74	45	35	48	33	12
Average	52	36	49	27	29	18
Total average	44		38		24	
Total downrange average			31			

* Height at which the rate of airflow was measured.

Table C7. Concentrations of lead on PBZ air samples of instructors

Date	Instructor ID	Sample Time (minutes)	Sample Concentration (µg/m³)	8-hour TWA Concentration (µg/m³)
	1	369	7.2	5.5
	2	373	5.5	4.3
	3	367	9.7	7.4
12/08/2009	4	357	11	8.2
	5	369	2.0	1.5
	6	359	(1.2)*	0.90
	7	86	ND†	—
	1	109	3.7	0.84
	3	414	(1.8)*	1.6
	4	254	6.1	3.2
12/09/2009	5	416	96	83‡
	6	243	ND†	—
	7	292	7.9	4.8
	8	241	ND†	—
	9	218	(1.2)*	0.55

*Concentrations between the MDC (0.61 µg/m³) and MQC (1.9 µg/m³) are listed in the table in parentheses to acknowledge that there is more uncertainty surrounding concentrations below the MQC.

†ND = not detected; the MDC was 0.61 µg/m³ for a 488-liter sample.

‡Exceeds the OELs of 50 µg/m³ for an 8-hour TWA; assumes no exposure for unsampled time during the work shift.

Table C8. Concentrations of lead on PBZ air samples of shooters

Date	Shooter Location	Sample Time (minutes)	Sample Concentration (µg/m³)	8-hour TWA Concentration (µg/m³)
	Lane 5	120	42	11
	Lane 8	145	340*	99*
	Lane 9	111	120	28
12/08/2009	Lane 13	108	56	13
	Lane 16	111	140	32†
	Lane 17	106	65	14
	Lane 20	109	55	12
	Lane 24	106	130	29
	Lane 9	121	58	15
12/09/2009	Lane 11	116	65	16
	Lane 14	102	49	10

*Exceeds the OELs of 50 µg/m³ for an 8-hour TWA; assumes no exposure for unsampled time.

†Above the OSHA AL (30 µg/m³); medical monitoring is required for employees exposed to airborne lead at or above the AL.

Appendix C: Tables
(continued)

Table C9. Concentrations of lead in general area air samples

Date	Location	Sample Time (minutes)	Sample Concentration (µg/m³)
12/08/2009	Staff Office	347	ND*
	Classroom	337	ND*
	Lunchroom	349	ND*
	Firearm cleaning area	343	ND*
	Firing range	347	(0.65)†
12/09/2009	Firearm cleaning area	413	(0.75)†
	Firing range – cleaning	138	ND*
	Firing range	364	3.6
12/10/2009	Firing range – cleaning	115	ND*

*ND = not detected; the MDC was 0.61 µg/m³ for a 488-liter sample.

†Concentrations between the MDC (0.61 µg/m³) and MQC (1.9 µg/m³) are listed in the table in parentheses to acknowledge that there is more uncertainty surrounding concentrations below the MQC.

Table C10. Concentrations of lead in floor vacuum samples collected on December 9, 2009

Location	Sample Concentration (µg/cm²)
Staff office	0.15
Front office	0.061
Safety supervisor's office	0.046
Front door rug	0.025
Lunchroom by front door	0.11
Lunchroom by computer workstations	0.071
Firearm cleaning area rug	0.24
Armory door rug	0.31

Table C11. Concentrations of lead in surface wipe samples collected on December 8, 2009

Location	Sample Concentration ($\mu g/cm^2$)
Staff office, first workstation behind computer	0.031
Front office, behind computer	0.11
Safety supervisors office, behind TV	0.12
Floor by facility front door	0.058
Floor by firing range door, outside	0.36
Floor, 10 feet behind lane 5	0.54
Floor, 10 feet behind lane 27/28	0.13
Classroom, table	0.019
Classroom, top of microwave	0.032
Lunchroom, middle of lunch table	0.026
Lunchroom, countertop near microwave	(0.0045)*
Lunchroom, top of modular cabinet	0.18
Lunchroom, modular desk by computers	ND†
Firearm cleaning area, left side front	0.085
Firearm cleaning area, right side back	0.17
Firearm cleaning area, top of filing cabinet	0.77
Firing Range, ammunition table 1	0.25
Firing Range, safety officer station	0.051
Firing Range, ammunition table 2	0.49
Armory shelving unit	2.0

*Concentrations between the MDC (0.004 $\mu g/cm^2$) and MQC (0.014 $\mu g/cm^2$) are listed in the table in parentheses to acknowledge that there is more uncertainty surrounding concentrations below the MQC.

†ND = not detected; below the MDC (0.004 $\mu g/cm^2$).

Table C12. Medical monitoring results, including BLL and ZPP of instructors (data obtained from an FOH contractor)

Instructor ID	Date	BLL µg/dL	ZPP µg/dL	Audiograms
1	03/2011	3	47	25 dB difference between left and right ear at 6000 Hz
	06/2010	<3	48	
	07/2009	3	28	
2	03/2011	6	39	
	06/2010	5	46	
	06/2008	5	48	
3	03/2011	<3	39	40 dB difference between left and right ear at 4000 Hz
	06/2010	5	56	
	07/2009	6	46	
	06/2008	5	49	
4	03/2011	3	36	
	06/2010	<3	47	
5	03/2011	<3	38	
6	06/2010	<3	45	15 dB decrement in right ear at 4000 Hz
	07/2009	<3	37	
	06/2008	<3	48	
7	06/2010	<3	44	
9	03/2011	<3	41	
	06/2010	<3	51	
	07/2009	<3	36	
10	06/2010	<3	51	50 dB decrement in left ear and 50 dB difference between left and right ear at 6000 Hz
	06/2007	4	---	
11	06/2010	---	---	20 dB difference between left and right ear at 6000 Hz

ACKNOWLEDGMENTS AND AVAILABILITY OF REPORT

The Hazard Evaluations and Technical Assistance Branch (HETAB) of the National Institute for Occupational Safety and Health (NIOSH) conducts field investigations of possible health hazards in the workplace. These investigations are conducted under the authority of Section 20(a)(6) of the Occupational Safety and Health Act of 1970, 29 U.S.C. 669(a)(6) which authorizes the Secretary of Health and Human Services, following a written request from any employer or authorized representative of employees, to determine whether any substance normally found in the place of employment has potentially toxic effects in such concentrations as used or found. HETAB also provides, upon request, technical and consultative assistance to federal, state, and local agencies; labor; industry; and other groups or individuals to control occupational health hazards and to prevent related trauma and disease.

Mention of any company or product does not constitute endorsement by NIOSH. In addition, citations to websites external to NIOSH do not constitute NIOSH endorsement of the sponsoring organizations or their programs or products. Furthermore, NIOSH is not responsible for the content of these websites. All Web addresses referenced in this document were accessible as of the publication date.

This report was prepared by Jessica G. Ramsey and R. Todd Niemeier of HETAB, Division of Surveillance, Hazard Evaluations and Field Studies. Industrial hygiene equipment and logistical support was provided by Donald Booher and Karl Feldmann. Health communication assistance was provided by Stefanie Evans. Editorial assistance was provided by Ellen Galloway. Desktop publishing was performed by Greg Hartle.

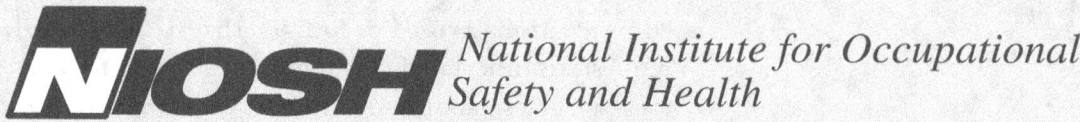

National Institute for Occupational Safety and Health

Delivering on the Nation's promise: Safety and health at work for all people through research and prevention.

To receive NIOSH documents or information about occupational safety and health topics, contact NIOSH at:

1-800-CDC-INFO (1-800-232-4636)

TTY: 1-888-232-6348

E-mail: cdcinfo@cdc.gov

or visit the NIOSH web site at: **www.cdc.gov/niosh**.

For a monthly update on news at NIOSH, subscribe to NIOSH eNews by visiting **www.cdc.gov/niosh/eNews**.

SAFER • HEALTHIER • PEOPLE™